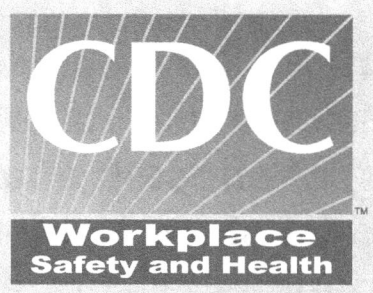

Ergonomic and Safety Climate Evaluation at a Brewery – Colorado

Jessica G. Ramsey, MS, CPE
Loren Tapp, MD, MS
Douglas Wiegand, PhD

Health Hazard Evaluation Report
HETA 2010-0008-3148
December 2011

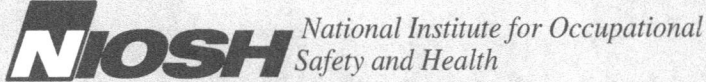

DEPARTMENT OF HEALTH AND HUMAN SERVICES
Centers for Disease Control and Prevention

National Institute for Occupational
Safety and Health

The employer shall post a copy of this report for a period of 30 calendar days at or near the workplace(s) of affected employees. The employer shall take steps to insure that the posted determinations are not altered, defaced, or covered by other material during such period. [37 FR 23640, November 7, 1972, as amended at 45 FR 2653, January 14, 1980].

CONTENTS

ABBREVIATIONS

HHE	Health hazard evaluation
MSD	Musculoskeletal disorder
NAICS	North American Industry Classification System
NIOSH	National Institute for Occupational Safety and Health
OSHA	Occupational Safety and Health Administration
WMSD	Work-related musculoskeletal disorder

HIGHLIGHTS OF THE NIOSH HEALTH HAZARD EVALUATION

The National Institute for Occupational Safety and Health (NIOSH) received a request for a health hazard evaluation at a brewery in Colorado. The union submitted the request because of concerns about musculoskeletal disorders. Tasks requiring repetitive motions on the can line and in the bottle depalletization (depal) areas were thought to be the cause of these disorders.

What NIOSH Did

- We visited the plant in January 2010.

- We observed and videotaped employees during routine work. This allowed us to document risk factors for work-related musculoskeletal disorders (WMSDs).

- We measured the heights of workstations and distances that employees reached to do a job task. These measurements determine the risk of injury.

- We talked with employees about their work, history of WMSDs, and their medical history.

- We reviewed occupational safety and health injury and illness logs. We also looked at employees' medical records.

- We asked employees about injury reporting behavior and perceptions of safety at the plant (i.e , safety climate).

What NIOSH Found

- Employees are at an increased risk for upper extremity WMSDs. This risk is due to awkward postures, forceful exertions, and repetitive motions.

- The rates of injuries and illnesses are similar to or below that of other plants in the brewery industry.

- Job rotation patterns were not consistent.

- The most common musculoskeletal injuries among can line and bottle depal employees were shoulder and wrist disorders.

- Employees indicated that safety training, policies, and procedures needed to be improved at the facility.

- Some employees felt uncomfortable reporting safety incidents or expressing their safety concerns. Employees felt the issues would either not be addressed by the employer or that reporting would result in a negative outcome, such as disciplinary action.

What Managers Can Do

- Design work areas to have a working height between 27"–62". Most lift tables should be redesigned so that the top rows are within this range.

- Add rotating platforms to the height-adjustable lifts.

- Rotate employees to different job tasks every break, instead of every 4 hours. All employees should use the same rotation pattern.

- Train employees on ergonomics and WMSDs. This will help them recognize and avoid risk factors that can lead to musculoskeletal problems.

- Encourage employees to report work-related musculoskeletal discomfort. These complaints should be logged to identify jobs that need to be modified.

- Keep employees informed about what is being done to respond to their health and safety concerns.

- Determine why some employees are not interested in efforts to improve safety in the workplace. Hiring a consultant with experience in this area may be useful.

What Employees Can Do

- Work safely and lift properly.

- Use the adjustable features on lift tables, platforms, chutes, and forklift trucks. This will allow you to be closer to equipment controls and the materials you are handling.

- Take part in safety and ergonomic committees.

- Report injuries and unsafe work conditions to your supervisor. You should also report them to the union.

- Seek care from a healthcare provider if you are injured at work. The provider should be experienced in occupational health.

SUMMARY

NIOSH evaluated ergonomic hazards, WMSDs, and safety climate among employees in the can line and bottle depal. We found that employees are exposed to risk factors for WMSDs to the upper extremities. Recommendations for reducing the risk of WMSDs include designing all work surfaces to be within a height range of 27"–62" and providing rotating platforms. We also recommended improving communication between employer and employees regarding employee safety and health concerns and encouraging employees to report work-related musculoskeletal discomfort.

On October 16, 2009, NIOSH received an HHE request from a union representative at a brewery in Colorado. The request concerned MSDs possibly caused by repetitive motions including lifting, pulling, pushing, and reaching in the can line and bottle depalletization (depal) areas.

During January 20–21, 2010, we visited the brewery. We observed workplace conditions and work processes and practices. We videotaped tasks on the can line and bottle depal. We also measured workstation heights and reach distances. We talked with employees privately to discuss their health and workplace concerns. We reviewed medical records of work injuries, and surveyed employees about their health and safety reporting behavior and perceptions of health and safety within the organization (i.e., safety climate).

We found that employees were exposed to a combination of risk factors for developing upper extremity WMSDs, including awkward postures, forceful exertions, and repetitive motions. Personal factors such as age, sex, smoking, physical activity, and strength can also influence the occurrence of MSDs. The employee interviews and review of OSHA Form 300 Logs of Work-Related Injuries and Illnesses confirmed that the most common WMSDs were to the upper extremity (shoulder and wrist). Twelve employees indicated they were injured on the job in the past 12 months; only half reported their injury(ies) to the employer.

Recommendations for reducing the risk of WMSDs include designing all work surfaces to be within a height range of 27"–62" and providing rotating platforms. The safety survey indicated that half of the employees feel that the safety training they receive is not adequate, and that the safety procedures and practices in place do not work. Recommendations for improving safety communication and involvement are also included in this report.

Keywords: NAICS 312120 (Breweries), brewery, ergonomics, can line, bottle depalletizer, shoulder, wrist, work-related musculoskeletal disorders, WMSDs, safety climate, safety reporting

Introduction

On October 16, 2009, NIOSH received an HHE request from a union representative at a brewery in Colorado to evaluate potential ergonomic hazards among employees. The request concerned MSDs possibly caused by repetitive motions during can line and bottle depalletizer (depal) job tasks.

During January 20–21, 2010, we visited the brewery. On January 20, 2010, we held an opening meeting with employer representatives, employee representatives, and union officials. We observed work processes, practices, and workplace conditions. We collected video of can line and bottle depal tasks and measured workstation design parameters. We also privately interviewed employees to discuss their health and workplace concerns, requested medical records related to WMSDs possibly caused or aggravated by repetitive work tasks, and surveyed employees with regard to health and safety reporting behavior and safety climate. On January 21, 2010, we held a closing meeting and provided preliminary recommendations to management and union officials. We sent a letter with our preliminary findings and recommendations on February 8, 2010.

Plant Description

The brewery was built in 1988 and included a 100-acre plant sitting on 1,200 acres of land. This brewery produced 8.7 million barrels of beer in 2009. Three can lines each produced 2,200 cans/minute, and three bottle lines each produced 1,200 bottles/minute. The plant employed 700 people including 83 employees in the bottle depal and can line areas. The plant ran 24 hours a day, 7 days a week, with 3 shifts. The plant had plant safety and departmental safety committees. Departmental communication meetings were held every 2 weeks, and a meeting with the general manager was held quarterly. The plant offered an annual ergonomic "Safety in Motion" training as well as peer-on-peer observations that varied in frequency by department. The company had two incentive programs, "Safety Beer," which provided a case of beer per person for every month without an OSHA recordable injury, and an optional wellness program that provided flexible spending account monies for nonsmokers who completed an annual physical and health risk assessment.

The brewery had an unstaffed medical clinic on site that was used for first aid treatment. If an employee sustained a non-emergency injury, the group manager was notified, and the employee was seen by the health and safety manager to determine if she/he needed medical care at one of the two local occupational medicine clinics contracted by the brewery. All employees were required to undergo baseline and annual hearing evaluations; emergency responders were also required to complete an annual respiratory questionnaire, respirator fit testing, and pulmonary function testing. The employer maintained OSHA Logs, injury/illness logs, incident reports, and workers' compensation records onsite.

Can Line

This plant had three can lines (61, 62, and 63). Following brewing and quality assurance, beer was placed into cans and packaged for distribution. All three can lines could run 2,000 cans per minute; the difference between the lines was how the cans were packaged. Line 61 handled only 12-ounce cans and packaged them in a 12 pack, a 6-pack Hi-Cone (cans held together with plastic rings), an 18 multipack, or a 24 multipack. Line 62 handled 12-ounce and 16-ounce cans and then packaged them in an 18 multipack, a 4 Hi-Cone, or a 6 Hi-Cone. Line 63 packaged 24 and 30 packs and a 24-pack suitcase.

We focused our observations on two tasks on the can line: filler and packer. The filler job on all three lines consisted of moving sleeves of can lids from an adjustable height pallet to an adjustable chute, removing the lids from the sleeves, and throwing the empty sleeves into a cart. While working on the filler job, employees also pulled cans from the line for quality control checks. We observed various packer jobs on the different lines; each consisted of manually placing cardboard trays and cartons of boxes onto the packaging line and disposing of empty pallets. While working on a packer, employees also performed quality control checks and were required to manually lift packs of beer. Employees rotated between filler, packer, and utility jobs in this department. Because of the variability of the tasks involved in the utility job, we did not observe this task. The rotation pattern in use during our visit required that an employee stay on the filler job for 4 hours. This was the only rotation that was mandatory; other rotations depended on the workgroup.

INTRODUCTION (CONTINUED)

Bottle Depal

We were asked to focus our observations in bottle depal on forklift truck drivers. Skids of empty beer bottles were received in trucks in the shipping/receiving department. Forklift truck drivers removed the skids from the delivery trucks and placed them on the depal line. A depal machine removed the bottles from the containers and sent them down the line to be filled. The drivers were required to keep two conveyor lines stocked, meaning they made multiple trips back and forth between trucks and the two lines. Additional tasks included cutting wrap from around skids of bottles and clearing jams in the machines. Approximately 4 months before our visit the company had implemented a rotation pattern where employees could only work on the bottle depal line for 4 hours. The other jobs in the rotation pattern were additional forklift truck tasks.

ASSESSMENT

We walked through the plant to observe the process of can line and bottle depal. We took videos to assess the tasks performed by the employees and measured workstation heights. While analyzing the videos of the work tasks after our site visit, we noticed that employees used visual display monitors at various workstations. The heights of the monitors were not recorded during our visit; however, recommendations are provided for heights that should eliminate neck flexion and extension. An optimal distance and position to eliminate reaching and elevated shoulder postures while using touch screen visual display monitors are provided.

We considered WMSDs as those MSDs to which the work environment and the performance of the work contribute significantly, or MSDs that are made worse or longer lasting by work conditions. A full description of the ergonomic evaluation criteria we used to determine risk factors for WMSDs is provided in the Appendix.

We held confidential interviews with employees working in the bottle depal and can line departments. The interviews focused on medical, occupational, family, and social histories. This included, but was not limited to, work type and duration, work-related injuries or illnesses, past or current health conditions, medications, and possible workplace exposures. We also reviewed medical records of employees who had WMSD symptoms, OSHA Logs for years 2007–2009, and company incident reports filed between December 2008 and March 2010. The incident reports were mailed to us after the site visit.

The employees who participated in the confidential medical interviews also met individually with a NIOSH project officer to complete a survey that explored work-related injuries and safety. Questions in the survey included injury reporting behavior; perceived consequences of reporting safety incidents and concerns; reasons for not reporting safety incidents and concerns; perceptions of safety climate; and safety knowledge, motivation, compliance, and participation.

RESULTS AND DISCUSSION

Ergonomics

Can Line

Filler

We observed employees working the filler job on Lines 61 and 63. Depending on the number of lids in the chute, employees performed four to eight lifts per minute. Each sleeve of lids weighed approximately 2 pounds. The heights and angles of the chutes were adjustable; however, it was unclear whether employees were adjusting the chutes. If the employees allowed the chute to become empty, they had to reach with their left shoulder abducted, sometimes leaning off the platform, to align the lids on the chute while removing them from the sleeve. If they tried to completely fill the chute, they had to either remove the lids from the sleeve with elevated shoulder postures or hold the sleeve with their elbow flexed for extended periods of time. The best option was to maintain the lids toward the middle of the chute. The height of the pallet of lid sleeves was adjustable but we did not see employees adjusting it.

Packer

Line 62 Multipacker

Employees used a vacuum lift to pick up two cartons of boxes at a time from a pallet located on a lift table. The cartons were stacked four high, four wide, and two deep. While the cartons of boxes were still on the vacuum lift, employees rotated them onto their sides and then placed them onto the machine conveyor. The lift table could not be rotated and employees had no room to move around the pallet, so they had to reach with their shoulder flexed to reach cartons on the back row. Once the cartons were on the conveyor, employees manually flipped the cartons over and allowed the boxes to slide out onto the machine conveyor. This required an awkward wrist posture during the flipping motion. The empty cartons were placed on top of the boxes until two or three were accumulated and were then thrown into a compactor. The height of the side of the compactor caused employees to have shoulder flexion during the throwing motion. When the pallet was empty, the employee lowered the lift table and slid the pallet off the table. A new pallet was then moved down a conveyor line onto the lift table. The lowest position of the lift table placed the top row of cartons at the higher end of the safe reach zone. Once every 10 minutes, the employee checked for defects by removing the cans from the case, inspecting them, placing them back in the case, and resealing the case. This required the employee to carry cases of beer as well as use a touch screen visual display monitor while reaching with elevated shoulder postures.

Hi-Cone Tray and 2-12 Packers

Employees removed cardboard trays from a pallet located on a lift table and placed them on the machine conveyor line. The height of the lift table could be somewhat adjusted but could not be rotated. Because the height could not be lowered enough, the reach to the top trays required elevated shoulder postures. Because the lift could not be rotated, the employee had to reach with his shoulder flexed for the trays at the back of the pallet. The video showed that the employee may have had room to step around to the side of the pallet to reduce the reach, but this action was not observed.

Line 63 Packer

Employees used a vacuum lift to pick up two cartons of boxes at a time from a pallet on a lift table. The cartons were stacked three high, two wide, and four deep. While the cartons of boxes were still on the vacuum lift, employees rotated them onto their sides and moved them to the machine conveyor. The position of the lift table required the employees to reach with their shoulder flexed for the boxes at the back of the pallet. The height of the lift table could be adjusted but not low enough for the highest carton to be in the middle of the safe reach zone. The lift could not be rotated; however, there was space to move around the lift, and employees were observed doing this to reduce the reach distance. Employees then flipped the cartons over and allowed the boxes to slide out onto the machine conveyor line. This required an awkward wrist posture during the flipping motion. The particular employee observed then broke down the cardboard cartons using the corner of the stair rail and threw them into a dumpster. The position of the dumpster and the fact that the cartons were broken down did not require as much shoulder flexion as the Line 62 multipacker. It was noted that vacuum lifts were available; however, they were not always used.

Bottle Depal

We observed one employee unloading pallets of empty beer bottles from multiple delivery trucks to two depal lines using a forklift truck. The forklift truck could move two pallets at a time. Occasionally, if a line was full, the employee removed the pallets from the truck and placed them next to the line because there was not room to place them on the conveyor. This resulted in double handling the pallets. The forklift truck was not equipped with rearview mirrors and did not have many adjustments. The placement of the computer caused awkward shoulder and elbow postures. Employees explained that they were responsible for unloading 8–10 trucks during their 4-hour rotation at this task. Each truck had approximately 38 pallets, meaning 304–380 moves per shift during this task. Employees explained that the other jobs in their rotation were more self-paced. Forklift operators were at an increased risk of MSDs due to prolonged sitting, trunk twisting and bending during reverse operations, awkward neck postures during reverse operations, and exposure to whole-body vibration [Waters et al. 2005].

Medical Assessment

Employee Interviews

We interviewed 36 employees during three shifts; 30 of 30 available can line employees, four of five bottle depal forklift operators, and two previous bottle depal or can line employees who had been transferred to different jobs for medical reasons. The 36 employees included 14 women, the average age of the employees was 48 years (range: 26 to 66 years), the average years working at the plant was 15 (range: 3 to 22 years), and the average time in their current work area was 9 years (range: 1 month to 22 years).

The interviewed employees were asked about current musculoskeletal symptoms potentially related to work tasks; nine (25%) reported having these symptoms. Eight of the nine employees' symptoms involved pain in the upper extremity, including four with pain in the shoulder, three in the wrist, and one in the thumb. Four reported that they had a prior shoulder disorder. Five reported seeing a physician within the past year for MSDs, and one had seen a physician 5 years before our visit. Two employees were on modified duty at the time of our visit; one had been on modified duty 4 months earlier. Four of the nine employees with symptoms stated they did not report their current MSD to their supervisor/employer. Seven worked primarily as fillers, packers, a combined filler/packer job, or as utility operators in can lines 61, 62, and 63; two worked in bottle depal. Six of the nine felt their symptoms were due to the packer job. The other three employees each named a different job they felt was responsible for their symptoms: the filler job, the utility operator job, and the bottle depal job.

Medical Record and Incident Report Review

Medical records of six employees were reviewed. Five employees had been diagnosed with a WMSD on the basis of their workers' compensation medical records; the sixth employee's records were from a personal medical provider whose notes did not discuss the relationship of the MSD to work. Four of six employee records involved shoulder pain; two employees were diagnosed with rotator cuff tears, one was diagnosed with pectoralis strain, and one was diagnosed with intermittent right shoulder pain subsequent to a prior shoulder injury requiring surgery. The other two employee records involved thumb, hand, and/or wrist pain; one employee was diagnosed with DeQuervain stenosing tenosynovitis, the other was diagnosed with bilateral thumb pain and mild deQuervain tenosynovitis. Two employees were waiting for approval to have surgery (one wrist and one shoulder) at the time of this review.

Eleven incident reports dated between December 2008 and March 2010 were reviewed. Three were initial incidents that led to medical evaluations included in the medical record review discussed above. The remaining eight incidents did not require a medical evaluation and involved five employees. Of these eight remaining reports, five concerned shoulder pain, two concerned wrist pain, and one concerned elbow pain.

OSHA Form 300 Logs of Work-Related Injuries and Illnesses

The results of the brewery's OSHA Logs for years 2007, 2008, and 2009 are described in Table 1. Sprain, strain, soreness, or inflammation entries were the most common and accounted for about 50% of all injuries in 2007 and 2008 but increased to 71% in 2009.

Table 1. OSHA Form 300 Log of Work-Related Injuries and Illnesses entries by type for years 2007–2009

	2007	2008	2009
Strain, sprain, soreness, inflammation	5	7	12
Laceration	1	5	1
Contusion/abrasion	1	0	2
Fracture	0	2	1
Amputation	1	0	0
Burn	0	1	0
Foreign body	1	0	0
Hearing loss	0	1	1
Total entries	9	16	17

Figure 1 describes these entries by joint type and shows that the shoulder was the most commonly involved part of the body and accounted for about 40% of sprain, strain, soreness, or inflammation entries in 2007 and 2008, but increased to nearly 60% in 2009. Job titles were entered for each of these shoulder injuries and included one administrator and one bottle line employee in 2007; one brewing, one can line, and one bottle line employee in 2008; and four can line, two fork truck, and one bottle line employee in 2009.

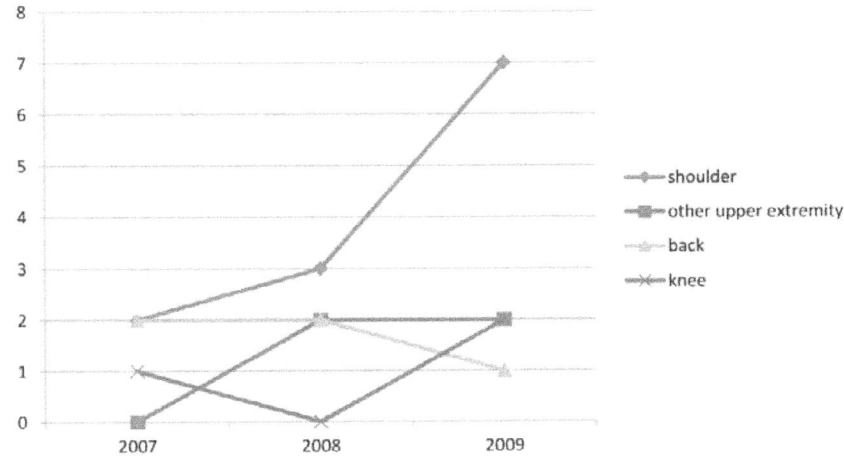

Figure 1. OSHA Form 300 Log of Work-Related Injuries and Illnesses entries for sprain, strain, soreness, or inflammation by joint type for years 2007–2009.

RESULTS AND DISCUSSION (CONTINUED)

We used data from the Colorado plant's OSHA Logs to calculate and compare incidence rates of nonfatal injury and illness between the Colorado plant and the U.S. brewery industry as a whole [http://data bls.gov/iirc/]. The incidence rates are for nonfatal injuries and illnesses per 100 full-time employees for each year (Table 2). These rates can be useful for determining problem areas and progress in preventing work-related injuries and illnesses and show comparisons across similar industries. These rates are calculated using the following formula:

Number of injuries and illnesses × 200,000 / employee hours worked = incidence rate

The 200,000 hours in the formula represents the equivalent of 100 employees working 40 hours a week, 50 weeks a year. From 2007 through 2009, employees at the Colorado plant averaged 41 work hours per week. Incidence rates in all categories would be slightly increased if the formula was modified to reflect this (using 205,000 hours in the numerator); however, we used the standard formula number of 200,000 hours to allow comparison to other plants with the same NAICS code throughout the United States.

Table 2. Comparison of nonfatal injury and illness incidence rates for years 2007–2009; Colorado plant (CO) and U.S. private industry plants with NAICS Code 312120 (U.S.)

Year	2007		2008		2009	
Case Type	U.S.	CO	U.S.	CO	U.S.	CO
Total*	4.3	1.4	3.9	2.6	3.6	3.3
Days away†	0.9	0.5	0.8	0.6	1.0	0.5
Job transfer‡	1.5	0.8	0.9	0.6	1.1	1.5
DART§	2.4	1.3	1.8	1.3	2.0	2.0

*total recordable nonfatal injury and illness cases

†cases involving days away from work

‡cases involving job transfer or restricted work activity only

§total cases involving days away from work (including days of restricted work activity and/or job transfer)

Incidence rates for nearly all categories at the Colorado plant are below the U.S. NAICS rates. However, from years 2007 to 2009, the Colorado plant shows an increase in the total injury and illness incidence rates, while the U.S. rates for this industry show a decrease. This increasing trend in injuries and illnesses during this time period may be due to an increase in reporting and documenting, or could indicate a real increase in injuries and illnesses.

Results and Discussion
(Continued)

The results of the medical interviews and reviews of medical records, incident reports, and OSHA Logs confirmed that WMSDs had occurred among bottle depal and can line employees, and that the most commonly reported injuries were to the shoulder and wrist. Review of the 3 years of OSHA Log data also revealed that the brewing department and bottle lines each had five musculoskeletal disorder entries during this time period. The OSHA Logs showed an increase in recordable WMSDs from 2007 through 2009, particularly shoulder disorders. Working at or above shoulder level, flipping material, prying, and pushing have strong associations with shoulder WMSDs. The combinations of work factors leading to neck/shoulder MSDs have been documented in previous studies [Holmstrom et al. 1992; NIOSH 1997; Miranda et al. 2001]. Personal factors such as age, sex, smoking, physical activity, and strength can also influence the occurrence of MSDs [NIOSH 1997]. In addition, rapid, repetitive hand motions have been associated with musculoskeletal disorders of the wrist and shoulder.

Safety Survey

Employees (n = 36) also met with us individually to complete a survey that explored safety reporting behavior and perceptions of safety within the organization (i.e , safety climate).

Work-related Injuries in the Past Year

Employees were asked whether they experienced injuries to their neck, shoulder, arm, hand, or back in the 2009 calendar year. Twelve employees (33.3%) indicated they experienced at least one of these injuries in the past year, for a total of 18 injuries overall. Hand injuries were the most common (n = 6; 33.3%), followed by injuries to the shoulder (n = 5; 27.8%), back (n = 3; 16.7%), "other body part" (n = 2; 11.1%), neck (n = 1; 5.6%), and arm (n = 1; 5.6%). Note that the results here do not necessarily match the responses in the medical interviews because of a difference in current symptoms of MSD (medical interview) versus acute injuries in the past 12 months (safety survey).

Of the 18 injuries reported in our survey, employees reported that 12 (66.7%) required first aid, six (33.3%) required a doctor's attention, five (27.8%) resulted in a job reassignment, and one (5.6%) was considered a lost time accident. Nine (50%) of these injuries were reported to the employer by six individuals.

Injury Reporting Behavior

As noted above, 12 employees indicated they had experienced at least one work-related injury in the 2009 calendar year. Six individuals did not report their injury(ies), five of these individuals reported their injury(ies), and one individual reported some but not all of his/her injuries.

Exploring Barriers to Reporting Safety Incidents or Concerns

Perceived Outcomes of Reporting a Safety Incident or Concern

Employees were asked if they reported a safety incident or concern (described as any injury, near miss, or safety hazard) they experienced or witnessed at work in the 2009 calendar year. Those who indicated that they had reported a safety incident or concern (n = 15) were presented with a list of possible perceived negative consequences they may have experienced as a result of reporting the incident/concern and were asked to check all that occurred. Ten of the 15 individuals (66.6%) selected one or more of the listed perceived outcomes.

The most frequently reported outcome (n = 4) was "the issue was not addressed by management." A small number of employees (ranging from 1 to 3) indicated they experienced either adverse job performance outcomes (e.g., disciplinary action) or poor interpersonal treatment (e.g., being ignored by others at work).

Reasons for Not Reporting a Safety Incident or Concern

Employees were also asked if they experienced a safety incident or concern (again, described as experiencing or witnessing an injury, near-miss, or hazard) in the 2009 calendar year but chose not to report it. Eleven participants (30.6%) indicated they had experienced a safety incident or concern, but chose not to report it. These individuals were presented with a list of possible reasons why they chose not to report the incident/concern, and were asked to check all that occurred.

The most common reasons were "I took care of the issue myself" (n = 6), "I felt uncomfortable about making a report" (n = 5), and "I thought I'd be labeled a 'troublemaker'" (n = 5). The other most frequently endorsed reasons (ranging from 1 to 3) included thinking it would make work unpleasant, not wanting to be questioned by the employer, believing nothing would be done to fix the problem, thinking the issue was not important enough to report, and concern over potential negative impact on one's performance evaluation.

Safety Climate

Safety climate refers to employees' perceptions of the safety-related aspects of their organization. One conceptualization of safety climate [Neal et al. 2000] focuses on individual perceptions of the value of safety within an organization, comprised of the following dimensions: *management values* (the extent to which the employer places a high priority on safety), *safety communication* (the extent to which an open exchange of information regarding safety exists), *safety training* (the extent to which training is accessible, relevant, and comprehensive), and *safety systems* (the extent to which safety policies and procedures are perceived to be effective in preventing safety incidents).

Employees' responses to the safety climate survey items were measured with a scale ranging from 1 ("strongly disagree") to 5 ("strongly agree"), with higher scores indicating a more positive perception of safety climate. Table 3 includes each safety climate survey item along with the proportion of employees who indicated agreement with the statement by scoring the question as either a 4 or 5 on the scale.

Overall, perceptions of safety climate were favorable among the employees. When summing the survey items into a comprehensive safety climate score, the average was 35 with a range of 10–50. Neutrality would be represented by a total of 30, indicating a neutral response of "3" for each of the 10 survey items, so an average of greater than 30 indicates that overall employees tended to view the safety climate favorably. However, examination of the percent agreement with individual survey items indicates that some areas need improvement.

RESULTS AND DISCUSSION (CONTINUED)

The safety climate dimensions with the relatively lowest scores were safety training and safety systems. Approximately half of the surveyed employees felt that the workplace safety and health training they received was inadequate and that they were not confident that the safety procedures and practices in the organization were effective. Another area of concern was safety communication, in which nearly half of surveyed employees believed they had insufficient opportunity to discuss and deal with safety issues in meetings.

Table 3. Proportion of 36 employees agreeing with safety climate items

Survey Item	Agreement n (%)
Management Values	
Management places a strong emphasis on workplace health and safety	26 (72.3)
Safety is given a high priority by management	21 (58.3)
Management considers safety to be important*	23 (65.7)
Safety Communication	
There is sufficient opportunity to discuss and deal with safety issues in meetings	19 (52.7)
There is open communication about safety issues within this workplace	24 (66.7)
Employees are regularly consulted about workplace health and safety issues	23 (63.9)
Safety Training	
Employees receive comprehensive training in workplace health and safety issues	18 (50)
Employees have sufficient access to workplace health and safety training programs	18 (50)
Safety Systems	
There are systematic procedures in place for preventing breakdowns in workplace safety	17 (47.3)
The safety procedures and practices in this organization are useful and effective	19 (52.7)

*Proportion of 35 employees agreeing with this safety climate item.

Safety Knowledge, Motivation, Compliance, and Participation

Participants were also asked individual-level questions to evaluate their safety knowledge, motivation to engage in safe behaviors and avoid at-risk behaviors, compliance with safety rules and procedures, and safety participation (i.e., supporting and promoting safety in the workplace). These survey items were measured with a scale ranging from 1 ("strongly disagree") to 5 ("strongly agree"), with higher scores indicating a more positive personal inclination towards safety. Table 4 includes each of these survey items along with the proportion of employees who indicated agreement with the statement by scoring the question as either a 4 or 5 on the scale.

RESULTS AND DISCUSSION (CONTINUED)

Of the individual-level safety dimensions, safety participation is the area that had relatively low scores, indicating that some employees did not voluntarily promote the safety program within the company.

Table 4. Proportion of 36 employees agreeing with individual-level safety items

Survey Item	Agreement n (%)
Safety Knowledge	
I know how to use safety equipment and standard work procedures	34 (94.5)
I know how to maintain or improve workplace health and safety	33 (91.7)
I know how to reduce the risk of accidents and incidents in the workplace	34 (94.5)
Safety Motivation	
I feel that it is worthwhile to put in effort to maintain or improve my personal safety	36 (100)
I feel that it is important to maintain safety at all times	36 (100)
I believe that it is important to reduce the risk of accidents and incidents in the workplace	36 (100)
Safety Compliance	
I use all the necessary safety equipment to do my job*	35 (100)
I use the correct safety procedures for carrying out my job	36 (100)
I ensure the highest levels of safety when I carry out my job	35 (97.2)
Safety Participation	
I promote the safety program within the organization	28 (77.8)
I put in extra effort to improve the safety of the workplace	31 (86.1)
I voluntarily carry out tasks or activities that help to improve workplace safety	23 (63.9)

*Proportion of 35 employees agreeing with this individual-level safety item.

CONCLUSIONS

Employees were exposed to a combination of risk factors for upper extremity WMSDs, including awkward postures (elevated shoulders and extended reaches), forceful exertions (lifting heavy weights), and repetitive motions (twisting and reaching). The overall rates of OSHA-reportable injuries and illnesses are below those of other plants in the brewery industry. However, we confirmed that WMSDs had occurred among bottle depal and can line employees, with shoulder and wrist injuries most commonly reported. The safety climate survey indicated that safety training and safety systems are areas that should be improved. Half of the employees surveyed felt the safety training and the safety practices and policies endorsed by the company were inadequate. This may also be reflected in the relatively low scores in safety participation, which may indicate that employees do not see potential benefits in promoting the company's safety program.

RECOMMENDATIONS

On the basis of our findings, we recommend the actions listed below to reduce the risk of WMSDs and create a more healthful workplace. We encourage the brewery to use the safety committees to discuss the recommendations in this report and develop an action plan. Those involved in the work can best set priorities and assess the feasibility of our recommendations for the specific situation at the plant.

Our recommendations are based on the hierarchy of controls approach. This approach groups actions by their likely effectiveness in reducing or removing hazards. In most cases, the preferred approach is to eliminate hazardous materials or processes and install engineering controls to reduce exposure or shield employees. Until such controls are in place, or if they are not effective or feasible, administrative measures and/or personal protective equipment may be needed.

Engineering Controls

Engineering controls reduce exposures to employees by removing the hazard from the process or placing a barrier between the hazard and the employee. Engineering controls are very effective at protecting employees without placing primary responsibility of implementation on the employee. Many of the height recommendations listed below were obtained from *The Handbook of Ergonomic Design Guidelines* [Humantech 2009].

RECOMMENDATIONS
(CONTINUED)

- Design all work surfaces to be within a height range of 27"–62". Moving the working height toward the middle of the range should reduce the risk for back and shoulder WMSDs.

- Provide lift tables with 36" of height adjustability.

- Redesign most lifts so that the top rows of lids, cartons, or trays are in the working range listed above.

- Use height-adjustable lifts with platforms that also rotate. This places the materials closer to the employee and reduces reach distances.

- Balance overhead tools (e.g., vacuum assists) at less than 74" above the standing surface.

- Place the top of adjustable visual display screens at a height of 58"–71" (adjustable height) or at 66" (fixed height). Place screens at a viewing distance of 18"–30" (adjustable distance) or 23" (fixed distance).

- Place touchscreen displays used while standing at a height of 47"–71" (adjustable height) or 59" (fixed height). Place the displays within a reach of 22". Tilt the screen slightly downward to avoid glare.

- Use rearview mirrors on forklifts to reduce neck strain.

- Provide industrial mats for employees who stand for 90% or more of their working hours. Mats should be ≥ 0.5" thick, have an optimal compressibility of 3%–4%, have beveled edges to minimize trip hazards, and be placed at least 8" under a workstation to prevent uneven standing surfaces. Mats can be ordered to meet specific electrical/static requirements.

- Implement a replacement schedule for mats. Mats should be replaced if they appear worn out or are damaged.

Administrative Controls

Administrative controls are management-dictated work practices and policies to reduce or prevent exposures to workplace hazards. The effectiveness of administrative changes in work practices for controlling workplace hazards is dependent on management commitment and employee acceptance. Regular monitoring and reinforcement are necessary to ensure that control policies and procedures are not circumvented in the name of convenience or production.

RECOMMENDATIONS (CONTINUED)

- Rotate employees through several jobs with different physical demands to reduce the stress on limbs and body regions. Rotate every break, rather than every 4 hours, to increase job variability. Use the same rotation pattern for all employees.

- Provide space around height adjustable platforms so employees can move closer to materials and reduce reach distances before lifting.

- Use a flat paddle or box grabber to move materials closer to employees and reduce reach distances before lifting.

- Investigate a way to remove boxes from cartons on the multipacker lines rather than flipping with the wrists; it may be possible to use the vacuum lift to tilt the cartons until the boxes come out.

- Evaluate the effectiveness of the implemented engineering and administrative controls.

- Schedule more breaks to allow for rest and recovery. Taking short breaks for 3–5 minutes every hour can give the body a rest and reduce discomfort.

- Train employees on adjustability features of their equipment and workspace and ensure that they are using them.

- Train employees on MSDs and ergonomics covering specific operations that have been identified by NIOSH or the company as causing or likely to cause MSDs.

- Perform surveillance with OSHA Logs and company injury/ illness logs to identify jobs that need intervention to reduce or eliminate ergonomic hazards. Our review of records indicates that evaluating the brewing department and bottle lines may be beneficial.

- Encourage employees to report symptoms of discomfort or pain associated with work tasks. Early reporting allows intervention measures to be implemented before the effects of a job problem worsen.

- Seek care from a medical provider with experience in occupational medicine if injured.

- Improve communication between the employer and employees regarding responses to employee safety and health concerns. A member of the safety management team should communicate directly with employees who report health and safety concerns to ensure the concern is understood and if applicable, what steps are being taken to address the issue.

RECOMMENDATIONS (CONTINUED)

- Consider hiring a consultant to help improve employee participation in the company's safety program. One area of focus should be to develop methods for encouraging safety reporting behavior as opposed to implementing disciplinary or otherwise negative consequences when such reports are received. The consultant may also be able to determine what the perceived weaknesses are in the workplace safety and health training so that improvements can be made to boost employees' confidence in the safety policies and procedures within the organization.

REFERENCES

Holmstrom EB, Lindell J, Moritz U [1992]. Low back and neck/shoulder pain in construction employees: occupational workload and psychosocial risk factors. Part 2: Relationship to neck and shoulder pain. Spine 17(6):672–677.

Humantech [2009]. The handbook of ergonomic design guidelines – Version 2.0. Ann Arbor, MI: Humantech, Inc.

Miranda H, Viikari-Juntura E, Martikainen R, Takala EP, Riihimäki H [2001]. A prospective study of work related factors and physical exercise as predictors of shoulder pain. Occup Environ Med 58(8):528–534.

Neal A, Griffin MA, Hart PM [2000]. The impact of organizational climate on safety climate and individual behavior. Safety Sci 34(1–3):99–109.

NIOSH [1997]. Musculoskeletal disorders and workplace factors: a critical review of epidemiologic evidence for work-related musculoskeletal disorders of the neck, upper extremity, and low back. Cincinnati, OH: U.S. Department of Health and Human Services, Centers for Disease Control and Prevention, National Institute for Occupational Safety and Health, (DHHS) Publication No. 97-141. [http://www.cdc.gov/niosh/docs/97-141/]. Date accessed: October 2011.

Waters T, Genaidy A, Deddens J, Barriera-Viruet H [2005]. Lower back disorders among forklift operators: an emerging occupational health problem? Am J Ind Med 47(4):333–340.

Musculoskeletal disorders are those conditions that involve the nerves, tendons, muscles, and supporting structures of the body. They can be characterized by chronic pain and limited mobility. WMSD refers to (1) musculoskeletal disorders to which the work environment and the performance of work contribute significantly, or (2) MSDs that are made worse or longer lasting by work conditions. A substantial body of data provides strong evidence of an association between MSDs and certain work-related factors (physical, work organizational, psychosocial, individual, and sociocultural). The multifactorial nature of MSDs requires a discussion of individual factors and how they are associated with WMSDs. Strong evidence shows that working groups with high levels of static contraction, prolonged static loads, or extreme working postures involving the neck/shoulder muscles are at increased risk for neck/shoulder MSDs [NIOSH 1997]. Further strong evidence shows job tasks that require a combination of risk factors (highly repetitious, forceful hand/wrist exertions) increase risk for hand/wrist tendonitis [NIOSH 1997]. Finally, strong evidence shows that low-back disorders are associated with work-related lifting and forceful movements [NIOSH 1997]. A number of personal factors can also influence the response to risk factors for MSDs: age, sex, smoking, physical activity, strength, and anthropometry. Although personal factors may affect an individual's susceptibility to overexertion injuries/disorders, studies conducted in high-risk industries show that the risk associated with personal factors is small compared to that associated with occupational exposures [NIOSH 1997].

In all cases, the preferred method for preventing and controlling WMSDs is to design jobs, workstations, tools, and other equipment to match the physiological, anatomical, and psychological characteristics and capabilities of the employee. Under these conditions, exposures to risk factors considered potentially hazardous are reduced or eliminated.

Workstation design should directly relate to the anatomical characteristics of the employee. Because a variety of employees may use a specific workstation, a range of work heights should be considered. On the basis of functional anthropometry, working heights should be within a range of 27" to no higher than 62" [Humantech 2009]. These heights correspond to hand height dimensions for the 5th percentile female and shoulder dimensions for the 95th percentile male.

References

Humantech [2009]. The handbook of ergonomic design guidelines – Version 2.0. Ann Arbor, MI: Humantech, Inc.

NIOSH [1997]. Musculoskeletal disorders and workplace factors: a critical review of epidemiologic evidence for work-related musculoskeletal disorders of the neck, upper extremity, and low back. Cincinnati, OH: U.S. Department of Health and Human Services, Centers for Disease Control and Prevention, National Institute for Occupational Safety and Health, (DHHS) Publication No. 97–141. [http://www.cdc.gov/niosh/docs/97-141/]. Date accessed: October 2011.

ACKNOWLEDGMENTS AND AVAILABILITY OF REPORT

The Hazard Evaluations and Technical Assistance Branch (HETAB) of the National Institute for Occupational Safety and Health (NIOSH) conducts field investigations of possible health hazards in the workplace. These investigations are conducted under the authority of Section 20(a)(6) of the Occupational Safety and Health Act of 1970, 29 U.S.C. 669(a)(6) which authorizes the Secretary of Health and Human Services, following a written request from any employer or authorized representative of employees, to determine whether any substance normally found in the place of employment has potentially toxic effects in such concentrations as used or found. HETAB also provides, upon request, technical and consultative assistance to federal, state, and local agencies; labor; industry; and other groups or individuals to control occupational health hazards and to prevent related trauma and disease.

Mention of any company or product does not constitute endorsement by NIOSH. In addition, citations to websites external to NIOSH do not constitute NIOSH endorsement of the sponsoring organizations or their programs or products. Furthermore, NIOSH is not responsible for the content of these websites. All Web addresses referenced in this document were accessible as of the publication date.

This report was prepared by Jessica G. Ramsey, Loren Tapp, and Douglas Wiegand of HETAB, Division of Surveillance, Hazard Evaluations and Field Studies. Industrial hygiene equipment and logistical support was provided by Donald Booher and Karl Feldmann. Health communication assistance was provided by Stefanie Evans. Editorial assistance was provided by Ellen Galloway. Desktop publishing was performed by Greg Hartle.

Copies of this report have been sent to employee and management representatives at the brewery, the state health department, and the Occupational Safety and Health Administration Regional Office. This report is not copyrighted and may be freely reproduced. The report may be viewed and printed at http://www.cdc.gov/niosh/hhe/. Copies may be purchased from the National Technical Information Service at 5825 Port Royal Road, Springfield, Virginia 22161.

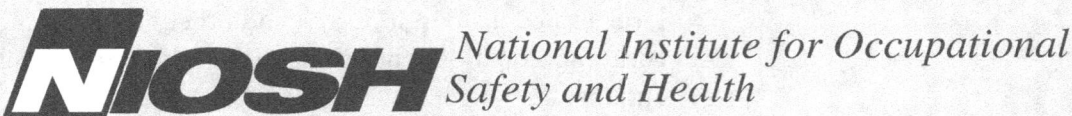

National Institute for Occupational Safety and Health

Delivering on the Nation's promise: Safety and health at work for all people through research and prevention.

To receive NIOSH documents or information about occupational safety and health topics, contact NIOSH at:

1-800-CDC-INFO (1-800-232-4636)

TTY: 1-888-232-6348

E-mail: cdcinfo@cdc.gov

or visit the NIOSH web site at: **www.cdc.gov/niosh.**

For a monthly update on news at NIOSH, subscribe to NIOSH eNews by visiting **www.cdc.gov/niosh/eNews.**

SAFER • HEALTHIER • PEOPLE™

www.ingramcontent.com/pod-product-compliance
Lightning Source LLC
Chambersburg PA
CBHW080941290526
45795CB00007BA/2847